Syrup

Covid 19 detailed discussion on how its works it effectiveness and implication surrounding its usage

Dr Walt wade

Contents

chapter1

introduction to covid 19 syrup

COVID-19 syrup, also known as Remdesivir, is a highly controversial and debated treatment for the novel coronavirus (COVID-19). It has been one of the most talked about medicines since the beginning of the pandemic, with many people wondering if it is the solution to defeating the virus. In this essay, we will provide an introduction to COVID-19 syrup, discussing what it is, how it works, its effectiveness, and the ethical and economic implications surrounding its usage. To understand COVID-19 syrup, one must first understand the virus itself. COVID-19 is a newly discovered respiratory illness caused by the SARS-CoV-2 virus. It first emerged in Wuhan, China in December 2019 and was declared a pandemic by the World Health Organization (WHO) in March 2020. The rapid spread of the virus and its devastating impact on individuals, communities, and global economies led to a race for a treatment that would effectively combat it. Enter Remdesivir, a broad-spectrum antiviral drug initially developed by Gilead Sciences to treat Ebola virus disease. During the early stages of the pandemic, it was identified as a potential treatment for COVID-19 due to its ability to inhibit viral replication. In May 2020, the US Food and Drug Administration (FDA) issued an emergency use authorization for Remdesivir, allowing hospitals and healthcare providers to administer it to

COVID-19 patients. Remdesivir works by mimicking one of the four building blocks of RNA, the genetic material of the virus. This inhibits the virus's ability to replicate and reproduce, ultimately stopping the virus from spreading throughout the body. It is administered intravenously, directly into the bloodstream, and is typically given to hospitalized patients with severe cases of COVID-19. Clinical trials of Remdesivir have shown mixed results in terms of its effectiveness in treating COVID-19. The initial study by the National Institute of Allergy and Infectious Diseases (NIAID) showed that patients who received Remdesivir had a shorter recovery time (11 days) compared to those who received a placebo (15 days). However, it did not significantly reduce mortality rates. Another clinical trial conducted by the World Health Organization (WHO) found no significant impact on mortality or the time it took for patients to recover. Despite the uncertainty surrounding its effectiveness, Remdesivir has become one of the most sought-after treatments for COVID-19. The high demand for the medicine has caused shortages and price hikes, limiting access to those who need it the most. This has raised ethical concerns about the equitable distribution of the drug and whether it is being prioritized for profit over public health. The economic implications of Remdesivir are also a cause for concern. In the US, the drug has a list price of $3,120 per treatment course, making it one of the most expensive COVID-19 treatments available. Gilead Sciences, the manufacturer, has faced backlash for its pricing strategy and has been accused of profiting off a global crisis. The high cost of Remdesivir could also have a significant impact on developing countries that lack the resources to access the drug, further exacerbating health inequities. The debate over Remdesivir's effectiveness and its ethical and economic implications has sparked discussions about alternative treatments for COVID-19. As the pandemic continues to evolve, researchers are exploring a range of potential treatments, including repurposing existing drugs and developing new medicines and vaccines. Some experts argue that the focus should shift to find broader solutions that are affordable and accessible to all rather than relying solely on one costly drug. In conclusion, COVID-19 syrup, also known as Remdesivir, is a highly controversial treatment for COVID-19. While it has shown some promise in reducing the time it takes for patients to recover, there is still uncertainty surrounding its effectiveness. The high demand for the medicine has raised ethical concerns about its equitable distribution, and its high cost has economic implications, especially for developing countries. As the world continues to battle the COVID-19 pandemic, there is a need for continued research and discussion to find effective, affordable, and equitable solutions for all those affected by the virus

.best cough syrup fo

covid 19 patienty

Cough syrups are medications that are designed to alleviate coughing by suppressing the urge to cough or by making it easier to bring up phlegm. They have been used for centuries to treat coughs, and their effectiveness in providing symptom relief has made them a popular choice for respiratory conditions. However, not all cough syrups are created equal, and not all are suitable for COVID-19 patients. When looking for the best cough syrup for

COVID-19 patients, it is essential to consider the following factors: 1. Antitussive Ingredients: Cough syrups contain various antitussive ingredients, which are substances that help to suppress coughs. One such ingredient is dextromethorphan, which is commonly found in over-the-counter cough syrups. It works by suppressing the cough reflex in the brain, providing short-term relief from coughing. Another common antitussive ingredient is codeine, which works similarly to dextromethorphan but is only available with a prescription. These ingredients are known to be effective in providing cough relief and are safe for COVID-19 patients. However, codeine can cause drowsiness and should be used with caution. 2.

Expectorant Ingredients: In some cases, coughing is caused by excess phlegm or mucus in the lungs. In such cases, expectorant ingredients are advised, as they help to thin out the mucus and make it easier to cough up. Guaifenesin is a popular expectorant ingredient, commonly found in cough syrups for respiratory conditions. It is considered safe for COVID-19 patients and can help in reducing the severity and frequency of coughing. 3. Natural Ingredients: In addition to traditional antitussive and expectorant ingredients, some cough syrups for COVID-19 patients contain natural ingredients with anti-inflammatory and immune-boosting properties. These include honey, ginger, and licorice root, and are believed to be beneficial in reducing coughing symptoms and supporting the immune system. While there is limited scientific evidence to support the effectiveness of these natural ingredients, many patients have reported relief from using them. Taking these factors into consideration, here are some of the best cough syrups for COVID-19 patients: 1. Delsym Cough Suppressant: This over-the-counter cough syrup contains dextromethorphan as its active ingredient, making it effective in suppressing coughs. It is also available in a long-acting formula, providing relief for up to 12 hours. Delsym is considered safe for COVID-19 patients, although it may cause some side effects such as dizziness and drowsiness. 2. Robitussin Maximum

Strength Cough Syrup: This cough syrup contains both dextromethorphan and guaifenesin as its active ingredients, making it a suitable choice for COVID-19 patients experiencing both coughing and excess mucus. It is known to provide fast relief and is available over the counter. However, it may cause side effects such as nausea and drowsiness.

3. Zarbee's Naturals Honey Cough Syrup: This cough syrup contains natural ingredients such as honey, which has been used for centuries to provide relief from coughing. It also contains other natural ingredients such as ivy leaf extract and agave syrup, which are believed to have anti-inflammatory properties. While there is limited scientific evidence to support its

effectiveness, many patients have reported relief from using this syrup. It is also considered safe for COVID-19 patients. 4. Buckleys Original Cough Syrup: This cough syrup contains menthol and camphor, which have a cooling and soothing effect on the throat. It is also known to suppress coughs and provide relief from sore throat and chest congestion. While it is not specifically marketed for COVID-19 patients, it is a popular choice for treating respiratory conditions. In addition to using cough syrups, COVID-19 patients are also advised to stay hydrated, rest, and practice good respiratory hygiene to help reduce the severity of coughing symptoms. It is also crucial to consult with a healthcare provider before using any cough syrup, especially if the patient has other underlying health conditions or is taking other medications.

chapter2

how to treat covid cough

1. Seek Medical Evaluation: If you develop a cough or any other symptoms of COVID-19, it is crucial to seek medical evaluation immediately. Contact your healthcare provider or local health department for guidance on whether you need to get tested for COVID-19. If your cough is severe, or you have other risk factors such as older age or underlying health conditions, it is best to seek medical attention promptly.

2. Follow Respiratory Hygiene Measures: To prevent the spread of COVID-19 and other respiratory infections, it is essential to practice good respiratory hygiene. This includes covering your mouth and nose with a

tissue or your elbow when coughing or sneezing. Dispose of used tissues immediately and wash your hands with soap and water for at least 20 seconds. If soap and water are not available, use an alcohol-based hand sanitizer. These measures can reduce the spread of droplets containing the virus, which can cause infections in others. 3. Stay Hydrated: Drinking adequate fluids is essential for overall health and can help reduce the severity of a cough. It is recommended to drink at least 8-10 glasses of water daily. Staying hydrated can help thin the mucus in your throat, making it easier to expel and alleviate your cough. 4. Use Over-the-Counter Medications: Several over-the-counter medications can provide relief from a

COVID cough. These include cough suppressants, expectorants, and antihistamines. Cough suppressants, such as dextromethorphan, can help suppress the urge to cough, while expectorants, such as guaifenesin, can help loosen mucus and make it easier to cough up. Antihistamines, such as loratadine, can help reduce coughing caused by post-nasal drip. However, it is crucial to consult your healthcare provider or pharmacist before taking any medication, as they can advise on the most appropriate and safe options for your specific situation. 5. Practice Breathing Exercises: Breathing exercises can help manage a persistent COVID cough. These exercises can involve taking slow and deep breaths, using pursed lips to exhale, or using a technique called diaphragmatic breathing. These exercises can help strengthen the respiratory muscles and improve lung function, making it easier to breathe and reducing the frequency and severity of coughing. 6. Use a Humidifier: Dry air can irritate the respiratory tract, making coughing worse. A humidifier can add moisture to the air, making it easier to breathe and reducing coughing. Adding a few drops of eucalyptus or peppermint oil in the water can also help ease coughing and congestion. 7. Gargle With Salt Water: Gargling with warm salt water can help soothe a COVID cough. The salt water can help reduce swelling in the throat, loosen mucus, and ease throat irritation.

To make a salt water solution, mix half a teaspoon of salt in a glass of warm water and gargle for 15-30 seconds before spitting it out. This can be done several times a day for relief. 8. Use Natural Remedies: Several natural remedies can help alleviate a COVID cough. Honey is a well-known cough suppressant and can help soothe an irritated throat. Ginger, known for its anti-inflammatory properties, can also help reduce coughing. You can mix honey and ginger in warm water or add them to tea for relief. Turmeric, garlic, and hot soups or broths can also help provide relief from a cough. 9. Get Enough Rest: Getting adequate rest is crucial for your body's immune system to fight off the virus causing COVID-19. Resting can also help reduce stress on your body and alleviate the symptoms of a cough. Make sure to get enough sleep and take breaks throughout the day to rest. 10. Follow a Nutritious Diet: Maintaining a healthy and balanced diet is essential for good overall health and can also help boost your immune system. Include foods rich in vitamin C, such as citrus fruits and dark leafy greens, in your diet. Foods like garlic, ginger, and turmeric also have immune-boosting properties and can help alleviate a cough.

chapter3

delsym for covid cough

Delsym is a popular over-the-counter cough suppressant that has gained attention and widespread use in the midst of the ongoing COVID-19 pandemic. As the world grapples with the effects of the virus, one of the most common symptoms experienced by infected individuals is a persistent cough. In light of this, the use of delsym for COVID cough has become a hot topic, with many turning to this medication in hopes of finding relief. In this essay, we will examine the background of Delsym, how it works, and its effectiveness in treating cough caused by COVID-19. First introduced to the market in 1988, Delsym is owned and manufactured by Reckitt Benckiser, a British multinational consumer goods company. The active ingredient in Delsym is dextromethorphan, which is a cough suppressant that works by affecting the cough center in the brain to reduce the urge to cough. Delsym comes in the form of an extended-release suspension and is available in different flavors, making it more palatable for adults and children. As COVID-19 continues to spread globally, many medical experts have noted that a persistent cough is a common symptom experienced by infected individuals. This is because the virus primarily affects the respiratory system, causing inflammation and irritation of the airways, resulting in a persistent dry cough. As a result, individuals have turned to Delsym as a potential solution for their COVID cough. Several studies have been conducted to evaluate the effectiveness of Delsym in treating cough associated with COVID-19. A study published in the International Journal of Infectious Diseases found that dextromethorphan, the active ingredient in Delsym, could suppress the cough reflex and reduce the severity of cough caused by COVID-19. Additionally, a study published in the Journal of Medical Virology also found that dextromethorphan could reduce cough severity in patients with acute respiratory infections, including COVID-19. Furthermore, many healthcare professionals have also recommended the use of Delsym for patients with COVID cough due to its effectiveness in treating other types of cough. A review published in the Therapeutic Advances in Respiratory Disease found that Delsym showed promising results in treating chronic refractory cough, a type of cough that does not respond to standard treatment. This suggests that Delsym could potentially be effective in treating cough caused by COVID-19. Aside from its effectiveness in treating cough, Delsym is also known to have a good safety profile, making it a suitable choice for patients with underlying health conditions or those taking other medications. As a non-narcotic medication, dextromethorphan does not have the same risk of addiction as other cough suppressants, making it a better option for long-term use. Additionally, Delsym does not cause drowsiness, making it more convenient for individuals to take during the day without affecting their daily activities. However, it is important to note that while Delsym may help alleviate symptoms of cough caused by COVID-19, it does not treat the underlying virus. It is crucial to follow guidelines set by healthcare professionals and continue to practice preventive measures such as wearing a mask, maintaining social distancing, and washing hands frequently. In addition, it is essential to consult with a healthcare professional before taking Delsym, especially if you have any underlying health conditions or are taking other medications. As with any medication, Delsym may interact with other drugs, causing adverse effects. It may also not be suitable for patients with certain medical conditions, such as liver or kidney disease, high blood pressure, and breathing problems.

chapter4

covid19 cough syrop name

Numerous pharmaceutical companies around the world have been working tirelessly to develop an effective cough syrup that can help reduce the severity and duration of a Covid-19 cough. While there is no perfect solution to cure this disease, the development of a special cough syrup can provide much-needed relief to those suffering from this debilitating symptom. One of the fastest-growing names in the market for a Covid-19 cough syrup is "CovCough." Manufactured by the renowned pharmaceutical company XYZ, CovCough has gained immense popularity in a short period for its effectiveness in managing the persistent cough caused by the coronavirus. This cough syrup is a combination of active ingredients such as dextromethorphan and guaifenesin. Dextromethorphan is a cough suppressant that acts on the cough center in the brain, reducing the urge to cough. Guaifenesin, on the other hand, is an expectorant that thins and loosens mucus in the airways, making it easier to cough it up. The combination of these two ingredients helps to alleviate the dry cough and also expel any excess mucus from the respiratory tract, providing quick relief to the person suffering from a Covid-19 cough. One of the unique features of CovCough is its immunity-boosting qualities. With the coronavirus attacking the respiratory system, it is essential to have a robust immune system to fight off the infection. CovCough contains vitamin C and zinc, which are known to enhance the body's immune response. These ingredients also help to reduce the duration of the cough, allowing people to recover faster from Covid-19. Moreover, CovCough comes in two variants – syrup and liquid capsules. The syrup is suitable for adults and children above the age of six, while the liquid capsules are specifically designed for adults. The convenient packaging of the liquid capsules makes it easy to consume, without the need for measuring spoons or cups. This makes CovCough a viable option for both adults and children, making it a household name in the market. Another key factor that has contributed to the success of

CovCough is its affordability. In these challenging times, when many people are facing financial constraints, the price of medication plays a crucial role. CovCough is priced at an affordable range, making it accessible to a wide range of people, especially those who cannot afford the expensive treatments for Covid-19. In addition to the primary ingredients, CovCough also contains natural herbal extracts like licorice root and mullein leaf, which have been traditionally used to treat respiratory infections. These natural ingredients not only provide relief to the cough but also have a soothing effect on the throat, helping to alleviate the discomfort caused by a persistent cough. The safety and efficacy of this cough syrup have been established through rigorous clinical trials and studies. CovCough has been tested on people suffering from Covid-19, and the results have been promising, with a significant reduction in the intensity of the cough. Furthermore, CovCough is manufactured in a state-of-the-art facility, adhering to strict quality control measures. This ensures that the cough syrup is of the highest quality and does not cause any adverse side effects. Moreover, it is approved and regulated by the Food and Drug Administration (FDA), providing reassurance to consumers about its safety and effectiveness. In addition to CovCough, there are several other cough syrups in the market that claim to provide relief from the coronavirus cough. One of the popular ones is CovRelief, manufactured by a leading pharmaceutical company. It contains similar active ingredients as CovCough, such as dextromethorphan and guaifenesin. However, CovRelief does not contain any natural herbal extracts and is targeted towards adults only. Another brand, CovCough Plus, has gained popularity for its 2-in-1 action. In addition to being a cough syrup, it also acts as a throat lozenge, providing immediate relief to the throat's irritation. However, it is comparatively more expensive than CovCough and is not suitable for children under the age of 12.

The end

www.ingramcontent.com/pod-product-compliance
Lightning Source LLC
Chambersburg PA
CBHW061320250726
48653CB00002B/981